De-stress Now!
Your Personal Program for
Reducing Stress

De-stress Now!
Your Personal Program for Reducing Stress

Dr. Ziggy Smith
BSc (Psych), Dip (Tra. & Ass.), Dip (FLM), M.P.E.T.,
A.P. Ph.D.

Oak and Mistletoe

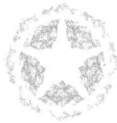

Oak and Mistletoe
PO Box 7393, Hutt Street, Adelaide, South Australia 5000
www.oakandmistletoe.com.au

First Published in 2008
De-stress Now! Your Personal Program for Reducing Stress
© 2008 by Ziggy Smith

National Library of Australia Cataloguing-in-Publication entry

Author: Smith, Ziggy, 1958-
Title: De-stress now! your personal program for reducing stress /
             Ziggy Smith.
ISBN: 9780980581805 (pbk.)
Notes: Includes index.
             Bibliography.
Subjects: Stress management.
             Stress (Psychology)--Prevention.
Dewey Number: 155.9042

For my students who teach me far more than I could ever teach them.

Table of Contents

Table of Figures

Foreword

This book arrived in my office amid a flurry of emails, paperwork, meetings and phone calls. It appeared as a message to me. How do I manage the stress of my working day? Do I successfully recognise those extra 'straws' that sometimes threaten to bring the load tumbling down, and then what actions do I take? Am I as 'in control' as I like to think I am? The relevance of the topic, and the promise of assistance, meant that *De-stress Now!* quickly jumped the queue to the top of my 'must read' list.

The program and information offered in this book will prove valuable to individuals and organisations alike. Some users will dip in and out, while others will do as I did and read cover to cover – then stop to reflect, before revisiting the sections most relevant to them at that moment.

For those involved in planning and facilitating workshops on stress management, this book provides an essential resource. The author's understanding of effective communication, group dynamics and adult learning are apparent in the carefully designed, yet flexible, tasks and triggers for discussion.

I commend this book to ….well, everyone. Whether you consider your days to be balanced or unbalanced, hectic or dull, relaxed or anxious, perfect or less than perfect, a tour through *De-stress* Now! is a very good thing!

Dr Kerri-Lee Harris
University of Melbourne

Introduction

The millennium cusp has been an incredible time for humanity. During the last fifty years, the planet Earth has been involved in one of the fastest periods of change ever experienced. Where once we were reliant on mechanical processes for productivity and wealth, now we're reliant on information and technology for the very same outcomes. The computer and access to global information in the blink of an eye means we can buy, sell, produce, swap, discuss, view, steal and create almost anything, with anyone, anywhere in the world. While that's given us greater freedom for the most part, it's also come with its own set of increasingly obvious headaches.

Rather than being the exception, stress is now the norm for many people in Australia and around the world regardless of their wealth, education, vocation or socio-economic standing. We work longer hours, we juggle more responsibilities, and we fight more battles, all with fewer resources, less time and often less reward. Australians now work some of the longest hours anywhere in the world. We've created our own stress epidemic that's damaging our workforce and our people so badly and we don't seem to be able to deal with it effectively. Part of the reason we may not be addressing the problem adequately lies in our very unique Australian culture.

Twenty-first century Australians inherited a culture that was born from frontier style challenges and 'making do'. Two hundred years ago, we conquered a tough and treacherous country with minimal resources and a fighting spirit. Against all the odds, we won the battle against the unforgiving, searing heat, the infertile, desert soil, the life threatening lack of water then dangerous torrential rains, the overwhelming distances and geographical isolation. We learnt that complaining didn't get us anywhere and that we just had to 'get on with it'. We became masters of creating new ways to deal with the difficulties and we were proud of our achievements. "She'll be right mate" became our cry of determination, pride and solidarity. Against all the odds, as a frontier people, we conquered our new world! Our universal saying served us well and it also helped us to believe we were completely self reliant, capable and resistant to stress.

While that self motivation and spirit continues to define us as Australians, it can also hinder us from seeking help when things go wrong emotionally due to stress or personal difficulties. For many, the inherent Australian pride makes us feel embarrassed to seek help. We feel we should be able to cope with problems as our forefathers did and that seeking help is simply a sign of weakness.

The other issue that many stressed people in the workforce face is the perceived consequences if their employer should realise they are stressed. Many of us worry about what the boss might say if we complain or discuss our feelings of stress. More and more Australians are employed in casual positions and even those in permanent jobs face the very real prospect of downsizing and redundancy. If we let the bosses know we're feeling stressed, then perhaps they'd just say "If you can't handle the job, I'll get someone who can". We may feel we run the risk of being overlooked for future promotion, having our hours cut back or being discriminated against for being 'weak'.

We get stressed as a result of elements that are often out of our control, but that stress is often dramatically increased when we feel unable to control or alleviate it. This might be due to embarrassment because the boss or colleagues might become aware of our situation or because of workplace pressure.

This major Australian program, De-stress Now! was designed to help people just like you by creating an opportunity for you to take control of your stress and conquer the issues without embarrassment or fear of the consequences. Because the program can be taken in the privacy of your own home, no-one ever needs to know your feelings, fears and concerns until or unless you want them too.

We all know that just 'sweeping it under the carpet' won't help to solve the problem in the long term. Sooner or later all that pent up aggravation, worry, tiredness and possibly fear is going to have an affect; and the result might not just affect you. Your partner, children, family, work colleagues and the boss are all going to be affected by the result in some way.

Instead of ignoring the issues, the most productive and effective way to deal with the problems of workplace stress is to bring them out from under the carpet, have a good long look at them and make informed and appropriate decisions about how best to deal with them. That's what this program, De-stress Now! is all about.

Because we're all individuals, this program is an in depth yet practical approach that will enable, and support you to identify and create your own strategies to effectively deal with workplace stress, or indeed stress in any area of your life. In other words, you'll be developing your own, personalised, tailor-made program, one that fits *you.*

Each one of us is different and this program recognises that. The program gives you the basic, simple to follow recipe of tools, you turn it into a masterpiece especially for *you*! By following the simple step by step processes on these pages, you'll have the practical tools and techniques to identify what stresses *you* and to reduce its negative impact on *your* life. *You* will back in control again! *You* can take charge of your life again!

So what powers will you master as a result of working through the tasks in this book? You'll be in control again and you'll be able to:

- Identify 5 factors that stress you so you can incorporate **better coping mechanisms,**
- Recognise your particular responses to stress so you can **feel better,**

- Find better ways to overcome stress so you can **channel negative energy into something more productive,**
- Find innovative ways to lessen stress factors so you are in **better control.**

How to Use This Book

De-stress Now! is made up of several chapters each covering a discrete but related element of stress. The program's designed to be progressive so that as you work through it, you'll be able to layer your new found skills and strengths to better cope with the stressors that are impact on your life. Although you can jump to a chapter that's an immediate need, the program works better if you start at the beginning and work your way through.

Throughout each chapter you'll find speciality text boxes. These boxes will highlight a certain point that will enhance your program by giving you some in-depth, tailor-made activities to really boost your program to get back into control.

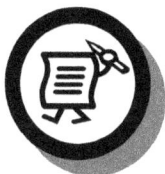

Personal Task

Within each chapter, you have the opportunity to get involved and take control of your stressful situations. Whenever you see this symbol, take some time to complete the task. By doing so, you give yourself a greater opportunity to experience a better way of dealing with stress by personalising De-stress Now! to meet your own needs.

Personal Task

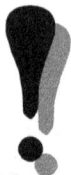

Important Note

You'll see this symbol several times throughout the book and it's worth taking extra note of what you read here. *Take Note* It's usually information that clarifies a point or reinstates something of importance that you need to take heed of.

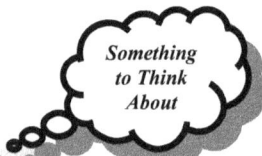

Something to Think About

You'll see this symbol several times throughout the book and it's worth taking extra note of what you read here. It's usually information that clarifies a point or reinstates something of importance that you need to take heed of.

So now that you know the layout of De-stress Now! Let's get stuck in so you can start creating your own personalised stress reduction program and conquer you issues of stress.

Common Stressors

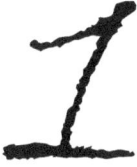

So you know you're stressed already otherwise you'd probably be doing something else right now instead of reading this. You can feel the stress in your body, in your head and in your approach to life. Some days it's not so bad, some days you should have stayed in bed. Some days you cope really well and wonder what the fuss was all about, other days everything's just one big nightmare. Know the feeling? Most of us do. The first question you need to ask yourself before you can snatch control back from the stress demons, is simple. What's causing you to feel stressed? In a nutshell, the answer's probably 'stress pollution'.

Stress pollution, put simply, is the sum total of all the stress you face each day, at work, at home and everywhere else come to that. But you stress pollution total is made up of individual 'stressors'.

Stressors are all around us, every day at work, play and with our family and friends. A stressor is any situation, event or process that causes excess stress and brings about a situation where you can no longer manage the issues effectively.

While everyone has different levels at which they no longer manage stress appropriately, different people are also affected by different stressors or causes. What one person perceives as being a major stressor, another could take in their stride. For instance, your work colleague laughs and shrugs off the nuisance of the photocopier not working today but for you, it's a major disaster and the final straw. They take it in their stride while you blow your top (or at least steam up silently in your workspace!)

There are some groups of people however who are often exposed to a greater level of stress than others may be. As collectives, these people are at greater risk of suffering from the negative impacts of stress. That doesn't mean they're guaranteed to blow their top when the photocopier malfunctions but it can mean that the constant level of increased pressure they face can impose on them a greater risk of a stress related reaction. Their stress pollution is much higher and like all forms of pollution, where it infects our lives excessively, there's usually a higher concentration of reaction. Some of those groups can be;

- People with limited or no social support networks report greater levels of stress than those who enjoy and use their support networks.

- Those who have a poor diet may be at greater risk of reporting stress related symptoms.
- People who are already suffering from a physiological illness or disease may experience greater stress levels than those who are physically fit and healthy.
- Socio-economically disadvantaged groups such as the homeless, unemployed, single parents or the disabled may be exposed to higher levels of negative stressors.
- Workers in known stressful occupations such as policing, fire-fighting and the military often report higher stress levels due to the physical dangers present in their workplace.
- Shift-workers and those who repeatedly travel through different time zones may have disrupted biological rhythms and so suffer from stress more frequently.

Now let's get something straight right now. Just because you're a policeman, a single parent or an international flight attendant doesn't automatically mean you'll suffer from stress related illnesses and repercussions. It simply means that people in these groups have additional stressors to deal with over and above normal workplace and daily life activities. Many people in those groups develop positive, healthy and appropriate coping mechanisms that enable them not just live through these situations but to actually thrive and grow from them.

There's also a considerable body of evidence that shows that both white collar and blue collar workers suffer from stress but that they report different stressors. White collar workers such as office employees argue that their roles and responsibilities, time management, travel commitments and work/home conflicts cause their stress. While blue collar workers like tradespeople and factory employees complain of stress for different reasons. They complain of work overload or in many cases boredom from not enough work or limited variety, poor work conditions and a lack of control and input into their job role.

Regardless of whether you fall into a predisposed group facing higher levels of stress pollution or not, there are still a number of stressors that can cause inappropriate stress reactions in the workplace and at home. Some of the most common stressors include;

- A difficult relationship with a supervisor
- Difficult relationships with co-workers
- Long hours
- Too heavy a workload
- Changes to the workplace
- Changes in role expectations
- Job insecurity
- Boring, repetitive work
- Harassment at work
- Workplace discrimination

- Crisis incidents such as accidents, burglaries or armed robberies in the workplace
- Insufficient or unsafe equipment to work effectively
- Limited skills for the job
- Poor workplace conditions
- Limited or no input into how the job should be done
- Lack of career development opportunities
- Lack of clear directions from management

No doubt you recognise some of these stressors if you're reading this book. You may be able to think of several other stressors that are affecting you instead, or even as well.

Stress can also be increased by stressors occurring at home, with friends or just about anywhere. For example driving can be very stressful particularly in rush hour city traffic. Perhaps your stress pollution also includes some of the following stressors;

- Marriage or partnership difficulties
- Illness of family members
- Financial worries
- Concern over the behaviour of teenage children
- Sleepless nights from waking infants
- Inadequate or depressing housing
- Bereavement

Studies show that it's not just the types of stressors that result in stress related illnesses and problems but it's also the number of stressors that you face at any one time. You might recognise only one or two stressors from this list but their impact on your life could be enormous. Alternatively, you may be experiencing the impact of a whole gamut of stressors. All those little things can add up to one giant dose of stress pollution just as one or two major stressors can be of equal damage in the stress pollution stakes. Whatever the combination of stressors, the result is excessive stress pollution infecting your right to a happy, peaceful, productive and positive life.

In the next chapter, we're going to look at a identifying exactly what stressors make up your stress pollution level. In addition, you'll use a common, highly regarded tool to define the amount of stress you may be facing so you can quantify it and measure it as you learn to cope with it.

The Social Readjustment Rating Scale

Readjustment: Adjust or adapt to a changed situation or environment (Concise Oxford English Dictionary)

One of the most common measurements of stress is the Social Readjustment Rating Scale (SRRS), designed by Dr. Holmes and Dr. Rahe back in 1967. Even though it's over forty years old, it's still a popular measure of stress.

Different stressors cause different levels of stress reactions and it's often helpful to know exactly how many stressors you face and what their total impact is likely to be. This scale attempts to define the impacts of differing stressors to give you a greater idea of how much stress you're actually under. So the SRRS lets you calculate your own stress pollution level, while at the same time helping you to identify exactly what stressors make up that pollution.

It separates the common stressors and rates them according to the average impact that it has on a person. The rating, or numerical value, reflects the degree of impact that you'd be exposed to as a result of the event. For example, if your spouse were to die, the impact would no doubt be enormous so the numerical value of that event is correspondingly high. As well as the obvious emotional torment, there'd be a series of issues that would also need to be dealt with that would increase the stress level further. These issues might include arranging the funeral, informing family and friends, sorting out the will and packing up the loved ones belongings.

By comparison, changing your eating habits would be far less stressful and so the numerical value of this event is quite low. You might go on a diet or decide to become a vegan and while the initial impact might be quite significant, it probably wouldn't leave you in such emotional turmoil as the death of a loved one.

If however your dietary change was necessary because of a serious illness, then there'd probably be a greater impact again. However, the SRRS would highlight the major illness as having one rating and in addition, you'd have another rating for the dietary change.

In other words, for each life event that you're experiencing, there's a rating on the scale that reflects the impact it might have on you. When you total the value of all these events up, it gives you an indicator about your likelihood of suffering from stress related problems and illnesses.

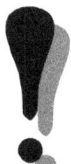

Important Note

It's important to remember one thing with this scale and others like it. Unless you're doing this exercise as part of a controlled stress program with a qualified practitioner, then you must make sure you see the result only as an average indicator. Everyone has different coping mechanisms for dealing with stress and those coping mechanisms will be more or less effective dependent on a number of life factors. We'll be discussing the changing tolerance levels of stressors in later chapters. For now, you need to remember that in isolation, the Social Readjustment Rating Scale is simply a tool to measure the average stress levels of the average person.

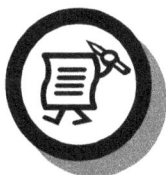

Take Note

Measuring Your Stress

Read through the list of Life Events on the Social Readjustment Rating Scale and circle the Value (the right hand column) of any Life Event that's happened to you recently. As you complete the list, remember there are no right or wrong answers. Where the Life Event says 'major change', this may be a significant increase or decrease in the subject.

Personal Task

When you've circled all the Values corresponding to the Life Events that have happened to you recently, total up your score at the bottom of the Value column. Then check your stress levels against those given in the 'Interpreting the Results' section.

Social Readjustment Rating Scale

#	Life Event	Value
1	Death of a spouse	100
2	Divorce	73
3	Marital separation from mate	65
4	Detention in jail or other institution	63
5	Death of a close family member	63
6	Major personal injury or illness	53
7	Getting married	50
8	Being fired at work	47
9	Marital reconciliation with mate	45
10	Retirement from work	45
11	Major change in health of a family member	44
12	Pregnancy	40
13	Sexual difficulties	39
14	Gaining a new family member (birth/adoption etc)	39
15	Major business readjustment (reorganisation)	39
16	Major change in financial state (worse or better)	38
17	Death of a close friend	37
18	Changing to a different line of work	36
19	Major change in number of arguments with spouse	35
20	Taking out a loan or mortgage for a major purchase	31
21	Foreclosure on a loan or mortgage	30

22	Major change in work responsibilities	29
23	A son or daughter leaving home for (marriage/university/travel)	29
24	Trouble with in-laws	29
25	Outstanding personal achievement	28
26	Spouse beginning or stopping work outside the home	26
27	Beginning or ceasing normal schooling	26
28	Major change in living conditions (renovations etc)	25
29	Revision of personal habits (dress, manners)	24
30	Trouble with your boss	23
31	Major change in working conditions or hours	20
32	Change in residence	20
33	Changing to a new school	20
34	Major change in the type or amount of recreation	19
35	Major change in church activities (more or less)	19
36	Major change in social activities (more or less)	18
37	Taking out a loan for a major appliance	17
38	Major change in sleeping habits	16
39	Major change in the number of family get-togethers	15
40	Major change in eating habits	15
41	Holiday	13
42	Christmas	12
43	Minor violation of the law (traffic ticket etc)	11
	Total	

Figure 1 Social Readjustment Rating Scale

Interpreting the Results

So now you should have a total that's a measure of your stress pollution right now. It's a snap shot of your stress pollution today and it's probably a good idea to redo the scale in a few weeks after you've taken some steps to reduce your stress levels and see if your total has dropped. Don't do it too frequently though, monthly is just fine.

Put simply, the higher you scored, the more you may be stressed. Please note though that I said *may* be stressed. Remember this is just a snapshot and it the results shouldn't be taken out of context. When Drs. Holmes and Rahe designed the table they determined that the following levels were apparent.

1 - 30

You're very calm, relaxed and trouble free. While this may be a comfort, you may not be living your life or working to your full potential. You may in fact be bored, lethargic, depressed or lonely and eventually that may contribute toward stress related outcomes later on, maybe not today but possibly at some point in the future.

40 – 70

This is the most productive range for stress management. At this level, you are probably working at your optimum level. Professional athletes and competitors aim for this level of stress to motivate them to higher levels of achievement.

A bit like the old sayings "All good things in moderation" and "A little bit of what you fancy does you good"!

80 - 100

If you scored in this bracket, you may be seriously stressed or at risk of suffering major repercussions from stress. You may be finding it extremely difficult to live life normally and your physical and mental health is at serious risk.

Your Score, Your Response

While this inventory has been one of the universal tools for stress identification for over forty years, it's only one of many. Research shows that just because you may score highly on the inventory, it doesn't necessarily mean you'll suffer stress in a predictable manner or at a predictable level. It's wise to remember this because otherwise you run the risk of falling into the self fulfilling prophecy dilemma. This notion says that if you believe calamity is around the corner, then sure enough, it will be. Remember, this is just a snap shot scale that you use as a tool to give you some pointers about stress levels at this particular time.

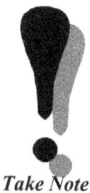

Important Note

Your response to stress is as individual as you are and dependent on many factors including your personality type, your historical ability to deal with stress and the

Take Note

range of stressors you are subjected to. Remember, always consult your doctor if you feel things have got out of control.

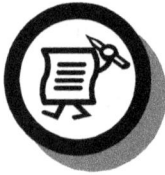

Your Stressors

Personal Task

Consider your own circumstances both at work and at home and think about the things that you believe cause you stress. By clearly identifying your stressors, you'll be better placed to recognise when they get out of control simply because you'll know what they are. You'll also be more able to reduce the implications of the stressors before they take control of you. In other words you're already taking control by being aware. We'll talk about this in the following pages but for now, use the Life Events suggestions in the Social Readjustment Rating Scale to help you identify what your highest rating stressors were and write them down on the next page. Your highest scoring stressors may be some of those suggested on the scale or they may be other equally as aggressive stressors that have a high impact on your ability to cope with life.

Write down the highest scoring stressors that make up the majority contributors to your stress pollution.

1 _____

2 _____

3 _____

4 _____

5 _____

6 _____

7 _____

8 _____

What is Stress?

3

The Concise Oxford English Dictionary describes stress as "a state of mental, emotional or other strain". Such a description would lead you to consider that all stress is bad. Actually that's not the case.

Too Much or Too Little Stress?

We all need a certain level of stress in our lives in order to operate at our personal best. Physical exercise places temporary stress on certain areas of the body and whilst we've all suffered from sore muscles because of over exertion at some point, regular exercise is known to be of long term benefit to the smooth running of the body.

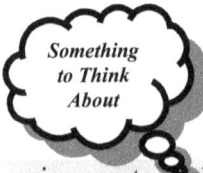

Something to Think About

Something to Think About

Mild temporary stress in the workplace can actually increase productivity and effectiveness, enjoyment and job satisfaction. Realistic but challenging deadlines often motivate us to complete a task on time rather than let it slide to the back burner. Special projects, challenging tasks, even exams can increase our productivity levels and raise our self confidence after we successfully complete the task.

In order to maintain healthy, mental stimulation and satisfactory physical fitness, the body must be exposed to a certain level of stress. For example, if you don't do any exercise at all, you may put weight on, increase your chance of illnesses, related aches and pains and decrease the strength of your muscles. If you do too much exercise at one time then you're highly likely to have very sore muscles the next day that you didn't even know you had! But if you maintain a regular healthy exercise program, your weight is more easily controlled, your muscles remain strong and your body agile and you generally feel much more healthy for far longer. You cope with colds and other virus and bacterial infections with greater success and you help keep yourself free from bone and muscle deterioration. In other words, a constant regime of appropriate exercise does you the power of good just like a constant regime of appropriate and optimum stress. This optimum stress exposure is known as 'eustress' and should actually be valued and encouraged.

When our brains are faced with a regular and constant situation without any stress, the result is boredom. When we live in a world without any appropriate and optimal stress we atrophy just like your muscles would without exercise. Un-stimulated and unchallenged, our boredom can lead to apathy, depression, withdrawal and in some circumstances, frustration-based destructiveness. Think about a time when you were so bored, perhaps at work or at a very boring party that just wasn't your style. How did you feel? Bored? Tired? Listless? Perhaps even fed up, angry or upset?

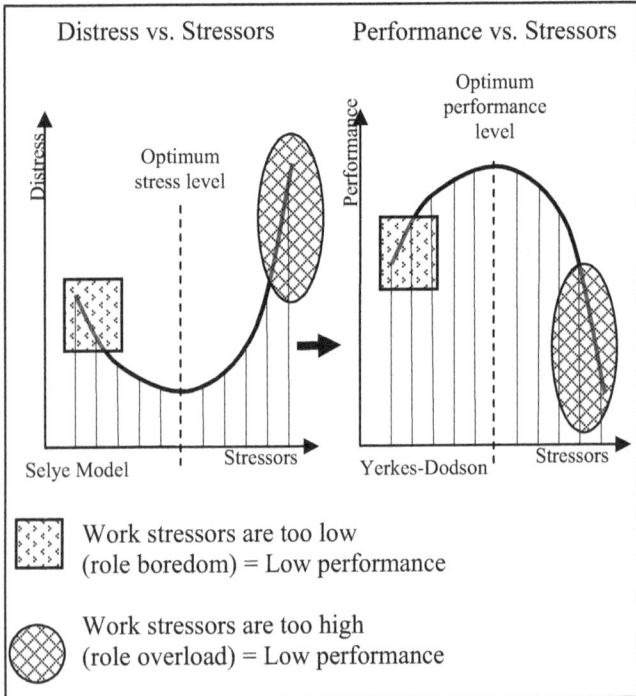

Figure 2 How Stress Affects Performance

Similarly when we're trying to cope with too much stress, we can collapse under the weight of that as well. Think of a time when there was just too much to d, and simply not enough time to complete it all. How did you feel then?

Overwhelmed? At a loss to set a plan? Worried if it would all work out properly?

Figure 2 helps to highlight the opposing areas of stress. When there's not enough stressors to stimulate us, distress is actually higher than it should be. We become bored, lethargic, unmotivated and maybe even destructive. Our work capacity decreases, our enjoyment of the job decreases and we exhibit the symptoms of being exposed to a stressful environment. If we're bored at home with nothing to do every day, we get fed up and sometimes become lazy TV junkies.

By comparison, when there are too many stressors, we are again subject to higher than normal levels of distress. We may feel overwhelmed, pressured, overworked and tired. Rather than working at our optimum level, our capability to succeed can be decreased as we succumb to excess pressure.

So what does all this mean? Put simply it means that if the stress level is too low, your performance at work and at home will be decreased because you're bored. If stress levels are too high, you're performance level is also decreased because there's just too much to cope with. Where there's enough stress to push us and stimulate us, (the vertical dotted line on the Distress vs. Stressor graph) our performance reaches its optimal level (the vertical dotted line on the Performance vs. Stressor graph).

As an example, in the early 1900s when some factories experienced significant decreases in productivity, the boredom faced by the factory workers who repeated the same task, on the same conveyor belt, day after day was found to be the primary cause. Similarly, many children who've been labelled as destructive or anti-social are in fact extremely intelligent and are simply suffering from mental boredom in the classroom. No one's stimulating them enough so they feel dissatisfied and without the maturity to cope, they lose the plot.

Let's turn from factory workers and kids to you now and look at what the graphs might show with your stressor and performance levels. I've illustrated possibilities using an X to show where the points of stress and performance might be.

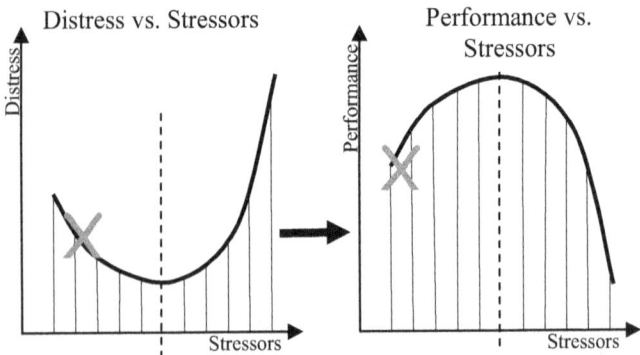

Figure 3 Not Enough Stimulation (Stressors) so Performance is Poor

In Figure 3 you can see that when there isn't enough stimulation, distress is higher than comfortable and the corresponding performance is usually at the low end of its scale.

Take a look at the look at Figure 4 and 5 to get an even better idea of how stress can affect your performance.

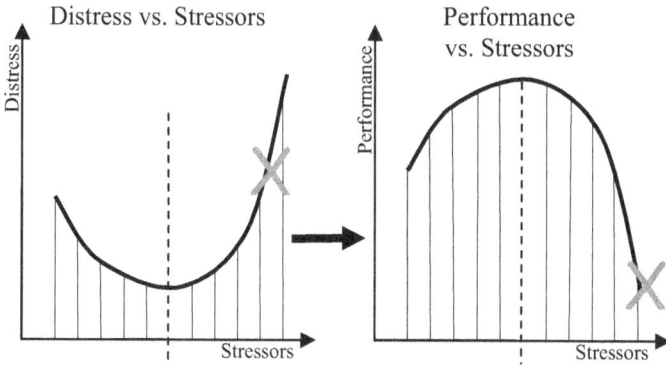

Figure 4 Too Much Pressure (Stressors) so Performance is Poor

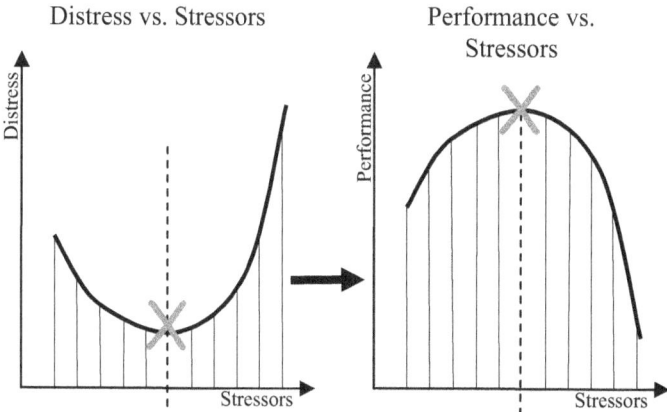

Figure 5 Optimal Pressure (Stressors) so Performance Peaks

By comparison, when there are too many stressors, distress becomes higher again while the performance decreases markedly in as a result.

However, when the stress level is at an optimal level, so too is the performance as you can see in Figure 5.

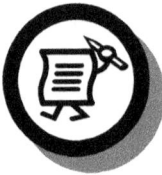

Defining Your Stress Levels

Personal Task

When trying to deal with stress related issues, it helps to know whether the distress you're feeling is caused because of a lack of pressure (not enough stressors) or because there's too much pressure (too many stressors). Consider your current status. Are there not enough or too many stressors?

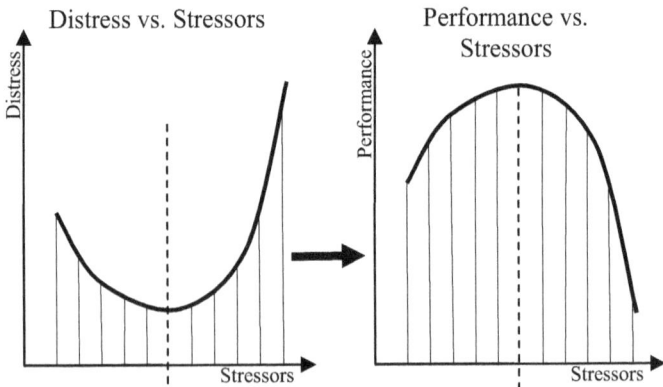

Figure 6 How Many Stressors do You Face and How Does it Affect Your Performance?

Take a few minutes to think about how much stimulation or pressure (stressors) have been placed on you these last few weeks. Have there been too few or too many? Would your X be at the low or high end of the Distress vs. Stressor scale? Knowing that, where would your X be in the Performance vs. Stressors scale? Place your X in the left hand graph in Figure 6 to indicate the level of stressors that impact on you.

Now that you've plotted the amount of stressors that you face, think about how your performance has been affected as a result. Chances are if your stressors are too high or too low, then your performance level might be on the low side. Plot your X on the right hand graph of Figure 6 to indicate your performance level.

You should now have a better idea of the stressor level that's affecting your performance and this information can guide you in overcoming the issues you face.

Tolerance of Stress

As well as differing levels of stressors, we're also affected by differing, but normal rhythms of life and these life rhythms can affect our tolerance of stress. These life rhythms include such events as adolescence, pregnancy, maturity, retirement and of course old age. For many women, premenstrual tension and menopause can be quite debilitating to stress tolerance. Men don't get out of this scott free either! Like women, they sometimes experience overwhelming pressure of early parenthood with constant sleep interruptions,

the emotional changes of fatherhood and the
pressure of full time work can also take its toll.
Men often suffer the 'male menopause' and when
the kids leave home, life often brings new
challenges and pressures for them as well as for
women.

Regardless of your gender, life rhythms
will have an effect on your ability to cope with
stress. Sometimes what would normally not be
stressful suddenly becomes a big issue, while at
other times, what would normally be extremely
stressful, is no longer a major problem.

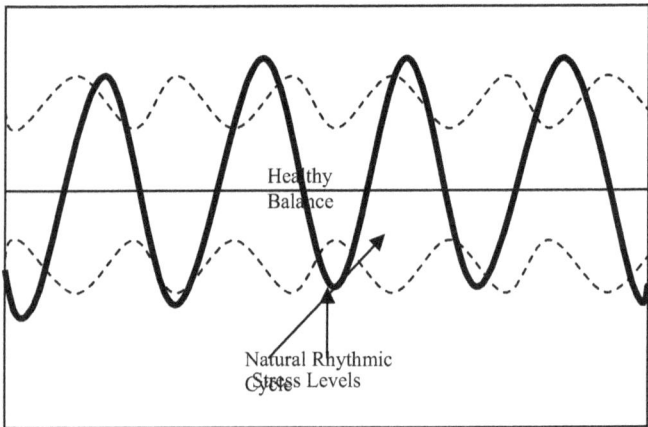

Figure 7 Changes to Stress

In Figure 7, we can see that stress levels
rise and fall just the same as the normal life
rhythms do. However, the peaks and troughs don't
always coincide so that on some occasions the
high stress peak might be present at a time when

the life rhythm is at its lowest. At that time, we may be less able to tolerate and cope with the stress. While at another time, the high stress peak may coincide with a peak in the life rhythm thus enabling us to tolerate and cope with it more easily.

Unhealthy Stress

While a certain level of stress is both necessary and healthy for productivity, motivation and physical and mental health, when the stress becomes overwhelming or we can no longer manage it properly, then we're said to be in 'distress', the opposite of 'eustress'. The stress pollution has finally become so overwhelming that we're no longer able to cope as effectively as normal.

What makes detecting or predicting stress so difficult is that each person reacts to situations based on their own personality and coping mechanisms so we're all different. There's no universal standard that can be applied to individuals to determine or predict their stress limits. People respond to differing situations in different ways so that what one person perceives as being highly stressful, another sees as being a stimulating and exciting challenge. Each person and each situation must be examined on its own merits. For you, that means that what upsets your work colleagues, your family or friends may not be upsetting to you or vice versa. What really pings you off leaves everyone else wondering what you're so upset about. Hence the need for a stress reduction program tailored just for your needs.

When the factors that produce stress (stressors) multiply in number or intensity so that someone is no longer able to control their responses or deal with the overwhelming situation, the body's ability to remain stable and balanced is impaired. This destabilisation increases the likelihood of stress related illness and reactions or inappropriate behaviour where actions are not taken to overcome the situation.

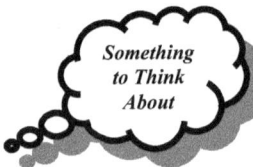

Something to Think About

Remember those destructive or anti-social children we discussed earlier? They may have capabilities well in advance of their peers but often don't get the appropriate attention and mental exercise and they may not have the maturity to manage their boredom. Without the appropriate social and reasoning skills, they may resort to destructive behaviour simply to release the pent up energy that hasn't been constructively and appropriately channelled.

What we see in Figure 8 is that when stress becomes overwhelming, our ability to tolerate it can often diminish in direct proportion to the amount of stress we're facing. As stress rises, our coping levels fall and further stress simply compounds the situation. At some point, the body and mind can no longer cope and they either succumb to illness or spiral into burnout.

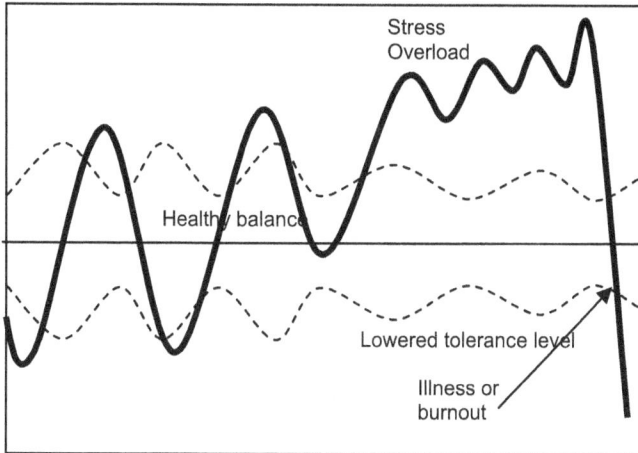

Figure 8 Too Much Stress

How Stress Affects Us

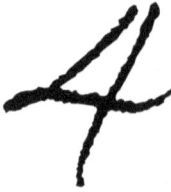

History Catching up with Us

It's interesting that even after so many millions of years of evolution, our bodies often still operate in ways they did way back when we were still living in caves and fighting for survival. The physical response to stress is one of those operations that continues to linger on from Neanderthal life right into our twenty first century existence.

Back when humans had to hunt for food and live in caves, they were often quite literally fighting for survival. When confronted by a hungry looking sabre tooth tiger, Neanderthal man didn't have a great deal of time to consider his options. He either had to attack the animal and hope he won so that he could feed himself and his family or run for his life! Put simply, when threatened his response was either 'fight or flight'.

Lots of changes occurred in his body when he was confronted by that dangerous, and probably hungry tiger. The brain understood that he was in serious danger so it sent messages to various parts of his body to get prepared for some quick action. The large muscles of his body needed to get hold of some extra energy quickly so that they could either fight the tiger or run away as quickly as possible. They expanded so that they could absorb more oxygen and energy to fuel their work. His liver pushed more sugar into the bloodstream and his breathing rate increased so that more oxygen could get through his lungs and into the blood. Then his heart started to pump much faster so that it could push that energy and oxygen rich blood through to the muscles that were preparing to work and conquer or flee.

Meanwhile, his digestive system stopped working so it could conserve energy for the muscles and his body started to sweat more so that it could more effectively cool itself. All this happened within a split second of seeing the tiger and realising he was in danger.

What was happening was that his body was responding to the threat by helping the leg and arm muscles to overcome the problem (fight) or escape from the danger (flight). When he'd killed the tiger or safely retreated, his muscles had used all the energy and oxygen they demanded and his body could then return to a normal state of operation. Good old Neanderthal man lived to see another day.

The problem with twenty-first century humans is that they're rarely confronted by sabre tooth tigers anymore and so rarely have to engage in a fight or flight response. Whilst some people are still confronted by a serious threat to their lives such as war or criminal assault, most of us will never have to face frequent physical threats everyday as our cave men ancestors once did.

However, our bodies still function as they did all those millions of years ago and they can't tell the difference between a physical life threatening event and an everyday stressful event. The body responds to all perceived threats in the same way it did all those millions of years ago. Essentially what this means is that the body doesn't really understand the difference between a threat at work and a threat from a sabre tooth tiger. It's stupid really but there you go!

What that means to you is that when you're faced with an angry customer at work, an ever increasing in-tray of work, a difficult colleague or another argument with a loved one at home, your brain thinks it's under threat and orders the body to go into fight or flight mode. Even that would be OK if you could get the muscles to do some work to use up the energy and oxygen they've created for themselves but our workplaces and homes aren't set up that way. Generally speaking it's not OK for you to fight the angry customer, run away from the overwhelming workload or beat up the loved ones at home. You're expected to continue as normal and 'get on with it'. As a result all that extra muscle energy is still there, the muscles are still tensed up ready for action, the digestive system is still on holiday and the sweat continues to run off your brow.

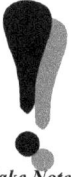

Important Note

If the body remains in this state, ready for fight or flight, for too long without an opportunity to release the increased energy and return to normal, it eventually goes into decline because it can no longer cope with the increased state of stress. Very quickly thereafter symptoms of stress begin to appear.

Take Note

Twenty-first Century Stress

Because each of us are unique and we all cope with situations differently, the symptoms of stress are equally as broad. The manifestation of stress can mask itself in illness or behavioural changes as well as generalised poor health. This variety of symptoms and disguised manifestation often makes it extremely difficult to pinpoint the true causes. While the manifestation may be physical, the cause may be stress related and initially unclear.

Broadly speaking, symptoms of stress fall into the three main categories of physical, psychological and behavioural. Some of the symptoms under those headings include;

Physical effects
- Headaches

- Sleeping difficulties
- Fatigue
- Heart palpitations
- Constipation
- Diarrhoea
- Heartburn
- Poor or reduced appetite
- Stiff or sore muscles
- High blood pressure
- Trembling
- Skin rashes
- Lots of colds

Psychological effects
- Feelings of anxiety
- Depression
- Confusion
- Aggression
- Inability to concentrate
- Crying
- Sexual dysfunction or disinterest
- Forgetfulness

Behavioural effects
- An increase in sick days or absenteeism
- A drop in work performance
- Angry outbursts
- Increased smoking
- Increased alcohol consumption

In addition to symptoms that can be clearly expressed to a doctor, counsellor, colleague, friend or family member, there's also the insidious symptoms that aren't so easy to describe. When suffering from overwhelming stress, many people complain of general feelings of tiredness or just feeling. They describe it as the feeling you get when you're 'coming down with something'. They may feel sad or not quite themselves but they're unable to fully describe why this might be or even exactly what the feelings are.

This general feeling of 'unbalance' is one of the main reasons why stress is so insidious and difficult to deal with in its early stages. Without clear descriptors, the cause can be somewhat mystifying. In the meantime, the cause (stressors) continue to mount and further unbalance us until more serious, yet preventable symptoms develop.

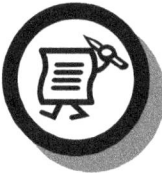

Personal Task

What are Your Stress Symptoms?
Take some time to think about your symptoms of stress. How do you behave? How does your body react? By noting how your body reacts or how you behave when stressed, you're better able to recognise these symptoms as they occur. This will give you a head start in dealing with the cause of stress before it gets out of control.

This unnoticed creeping up of symptoms is a real danger of stress. Stress pollution can mount up like fog on a cold morning. Before you know it, you're so engulfed in the misty swirls around you that you can't see where you're going anymore. Stress pollution is the same. Your best defence as a starting point is to observe your responses and use them as a signpost that the stress levels are beginning to creep up too quickly like that fog.

In addition, by identifying whether the reaction is physical, psychological or behavioural, it will also give you an indication of the best way to tackle the reactions. Each type of stress reaction will probably require a slightly different approach so if you can identify the type of reaction to stress that you manifest, you're in a much better position to define the best way to deal with it.

Physical	Psychological	Behavioural

On the table on the previous page, write down as many stress reactions as you can that you experience under the three headings. You may find that your reactions fall mainly in one area, or they may be spread across all three areas.

Eliminating or Reducing Stressors

5

> *Success: The accomplishment of an aim or purpose (Concise Oxford English Dictionary)*

Up to this point you've identified the causes of your stress, recognised how you react to stress and now it's time to design some ways to eliminate or overcome some of those stressors.

When we're feeling particularly stressed and at a loss to deal with life's dilemmas, we often dream of a stress free life with no major responsibilities and no disruptive relationships to sour the ideal. Then reality comes along quite abruptly and hits us squarely on the chin.

The first lesson we need to learn is that we're never going to be in a totally stress free life. We've already learnt that in fact we need some degree of appropriate stress in order to perform at our optimal level. Having said that, when the stress pollution starts taking over, that's when we have to start making some decisions and work our way back into the clean air again.

In everyday life there are some stressors we can control and there are some we just have to learn to live with. The trick is to identify which ones we can control and either reduce or eliminate them, and which ones we just have to learn to live with more effectively. We can't control the idiot driver who cuts us off but we can control our input to our marriages or family life. Take a look at this list of common stressors according to our ability to be control them or otherwise.

Stressors we can control
- Too many phone calls
- Taking on too much work
- Not enough skills for the job
- Too many hours at work
- Too many interruptions
- Harassment at work
- Discrimination at work
- Not enough work to do
- Too many emails
- Financial difficulties
- Marriage problems

Stressors we can't control
- Too much peak hour traffic
- Predetermined deadlines
- Angry customers
- Limited variety in the job
- Crisis incidents
- Difficult work colleagues
- Difficult supervisor
- Job insecurity
- No career prospects

- Family illnesses
- Death of a friend or family member

Depending on your workplace, your circumstances at home, your personality type and your methods of coping, some of these stressors may in fact need to swap from controllable to uncontrollable or vice versa. For instance, in this illustration 'too many hours at work' fits under the stressors that can be controlled. For many people, they can make the choice to reduce the hours spent at work. However, you might work in an environment where, temporarily or permanently, you simply aren't in a position to reduce your hours. This may be because there's a special project occurring for which there's a deadline and other than leaving your job, it simply must be done. On the other hand, the stressor, 'too much peak hour traffic' fits under the uncontrollable stressors because most people need to arrive and leave work at set times. For some people though, it may be possible to negotiate different start and finishing times so that traffic delays are no longer a concern. Perhaps you could come in an hour later and stay an hour later at night.

At home, there are different stressors. You could suggest that you can't control when the washing machine breaks down or when the kids get ill but in fact you might be able to control when the washing machine gets fixed and how quickly you can get the kids to a doctor. The point is to determine what your stressors are and to then decide how much control you have over each of them.

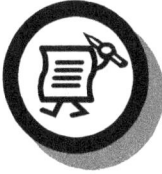

Controllable and Uncontrollable Stressors

Now it's time to work out how much control you have over the stressors in *your* life. In the table in Figure 9, write down all the stressors that have an impact on your life. Place them in the table according to their level of control.

For example, if you find an excess of emails frustrating but there's nothing you can do about it, then it goes in the right column under 'Stressors I need to learn to cope with'. If you get frustrated because you don't have all the skills you feel you need for your job and you are able to do something
about it, then it fits into the other column instead. Think carefully and capture all the stressors you can.

Take your time to think about all the stressors that affect you every day. Think about the stressors at work, at home and socially. Stressors come in all shapes and sizes and many different areas of our lives. The stressors that make up your stress pollution could come from a variety of sources.

When you begin this exercise, it may seem that many of the stressors fir into the right hand column where you have no control over them.

This can seem a little daunting at first but in later chapters, you'll find some tools that might empower you to actually take control of some of those stressors too. Many workplaces now offer flexible options to help you come to grips with issues that affect your performance levels. With a rational discussion with your manager and a well thought out proposition to increase your own productivity, you may be in a prime position to negotiate changes that enable you to work better and reduce stress, even those stressors you thought were out of your control.

Stressors I can eliminate or reduce	Stressors I need to learn to cope with

Figure 9 Stressor Control

Now you have a list of issues that cause you continued stress but you're also able to identify those that can be eliminated or reduced. We'll deal with the uncontrollable stressors in the next chapter but for now, let's concentrate on those ones you can do something about.

Some of these stressors could be reduced quite quickly. Although quick-win solutions will obviously be dependent upon the problem, some common reduction strategies include;

- Shutting your office door at least for part of the day to reduce personal interruptions,
- Masking your workstation with pot plants to make it a more peaceful environment and to hide it from potential interruptions,
- Bringing in some family photos to make your workplace more personal,
- Learning how to say "no" so that you don't take on more work than you cope with,
- Putting your phone onto message bank for one hour each day so that you can work undisturbed for a period,
- Setting 'me' time at home away from the kids to refresh yourself.

Some measures might take a little longer to achieve. These might include;

- Making a joint agreement with the boss to improve the relationship so that you can both work more effectively together,
- Working with management to design a better role description so that you feel more fulfilled and satisfied,
- Doing some additional skills training in the areas you feel less confident in to help you become more productive,

- Organising to go to a meditation class.

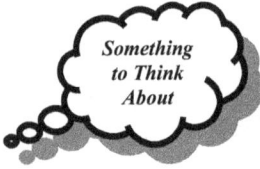

Something to Think About

The trick here is to think about the stressors differently from the way you've seen them before. Up until now, you've probably considered these issues a nuisance, the absolute pain of your life, a bunch of soul destroying issues that ruin your days. Yes, of course they're a pain but now that you've isolated them as issues you can control, you can begin to think of ways to control them.

One easy way to do this is to brainstorm possible solutions. Take a blank piece of paper and at the top write down the stressor. Then underneath, think of all the ways you could control it through elimination or reduction. Be creative, be outrageous, make your ideas as wacky and off the wall as you like. Don't qualify any ideas at this point. Even if the solutions seem utterly ridiculous, write them down. Creative and workable solutions often come from the unexpected.

When you've exhausted all your possible solutions, then you can begin to look at them to see what will work and what won't. Of the ones that might work, number them in order of how effective you think they might be and then give them a try! Let's have a practice.

Our example stressor is 'not enough desk space'. With that title at the top of our paper, write down all the ways you could overcome that. Remember to let the wacky and obviously unusable ideas flow too. It doesn't matter if the ideas seem ridiculous, let them come. They might lead you in a direction that gives you the best answer.

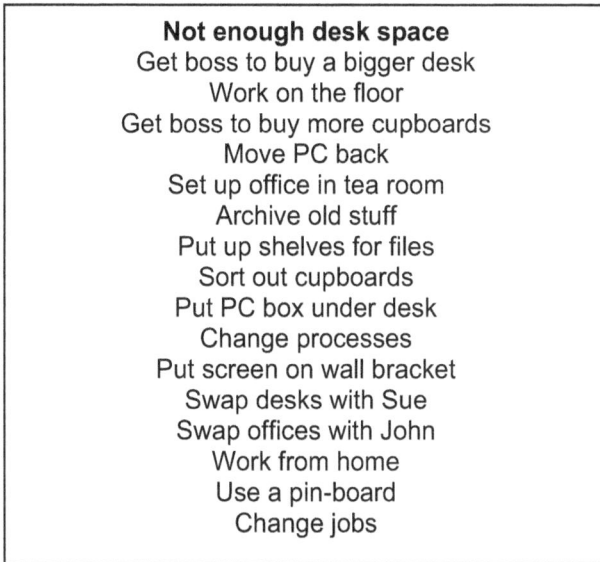

Not enough desk space
Get boss to buy a bigger desk
Work on the floor
Get boss to buy more cupboards
Move PC back
Set up office in tea room
Archive old stuff
Put up shelves for files
Sort out cupboards
Put PC box under desk
Change processes
Put screen on wall bracket
Swap desks with Sue
Swap offices with John
Work from home
Use a pin-board
Change jobs

Figure 10 Stressor Brainstorm 1

Now you can begin to throw out the ideas you know won't work. They served you well in helping the flow of creativity but now you need to get serious. You need to get a little closer to the ideas that will be more useful in reality. Look at the ideas again and draw a line through those ones that seem impractical or far too difficult to implement for some reason. Having done that, your page might look more like Figure 11.

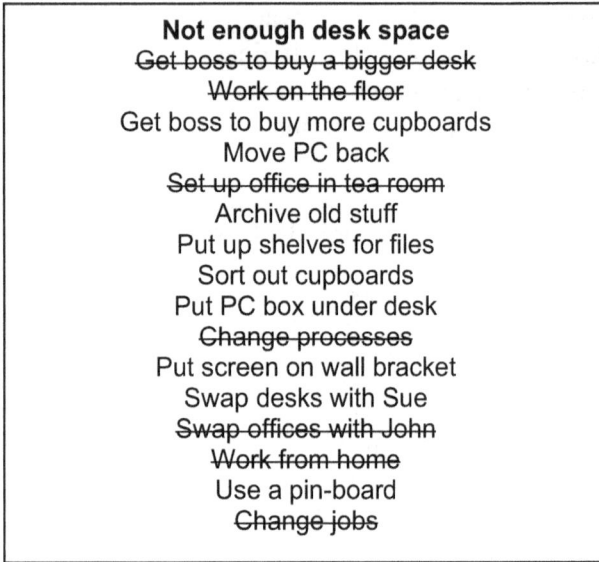

Not enough desk space
~~Get boss to buy a bigger desk~~
~~Work on the floor~~
Get boss to buy more cupboards
Move PC back
~~Set up office in tea room~~
Archive old stuff
Put up shelves for files
Sort out cupboards
Put PC box under desk
~~Change processes~~
Put screen on wall bracket
Swap desks with Sue
~~Swap offices with John~~
~~Work from home~~
Use a pin-board
~~Change jobs~~

Figure 11 Stressor Brainstorm 2

The last task is to put the remaining ideas into an order of preference with the most workable as number 1. This is the stage where you really begin to think about which ideas have more value than others. You may even have to implement one idea before you use the next. For example, you may not be able to archive the old material until you've sorted out the cupboards. Hence sorting the cupboards is rated number 1 while the archiving is rated at number 2.

You may also find at this time that you have a series of ideas that can work simultaneously or one can be a back-up idea if another doesn't quite work. For instance you might be able to put the PC box under the table as well as put up more shelves. Or you may have to resort to putting the PC box under the desk if you can't put shelves up for your files.

This is also the rewarding stage as you now have a battle plan for dealing with the problems that have been bugging you for so long. Your page finally might look similar to Figure 12 with some numbered priorities and clear direction emerging.

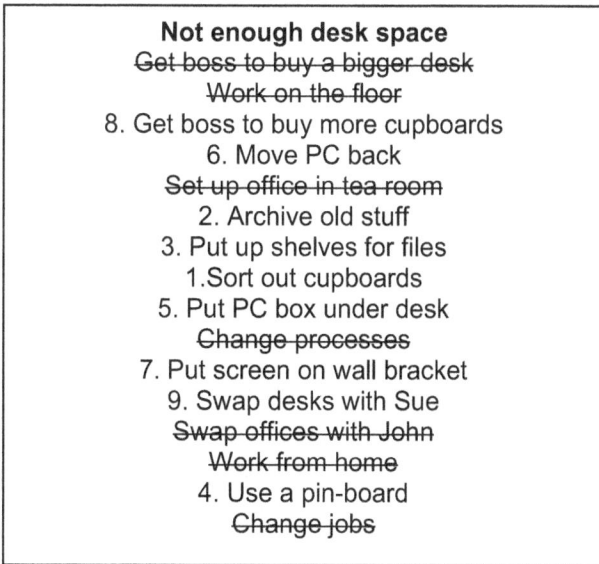

Not enough desk space
~~Get boss to buy a bigger desk~~
~~Work on the floor~~
8. Get boss to buy more cupboards
6. Move PC back
~~Set up office in tea room~~
2. Archive old stuff
3. Put up shelves for files
1.Sort out cupboards
5. Put PC box under desk
~~Change processes~~
7. Put screen on wall bracket
9. Swap desks with Sue
~~Swap offices with John~~
~~Work from home~~
4. Use a pin-board
~~Change jobs~~

Figure 12 Stressor Brainstorm 3

Now you really have the beginnings of your own tailor-made, personalised stress reduction plan! You've taken control of the issue and you've worked out how to begin the process of controlling the stressor that was causing you so many difficulties. You created the plan!

With that done, your next task is to actually implement the plan. First we'll sort out the existing cupboards and then archive the old material. From there, we'll put up the shelves for the files and so on.

What you've actually done is design a plan to tackle the stressor and then put it into action. The plan has its own built in alternatives if the first option doesn't work and it lists in order of preference the best way to handle the problem. Congratulations, you did it!

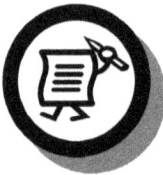

Taking Steps to Eliminate or Reduce Stressors in Your Workplace

Personal Task

Now it's time to take your level of control another step further. Transfer the controllable stressors you wrote down in the last Personal Task to the left column of the table in Figure 13 . Take a blank sheet of paper and some coloured pens and get your creative juices flowing again. With that list of controllable stressors, brainstorm all the solutions you can think of, both workable and the ridiculous, 'off the wall' ones.

Take your time, be creative, feed ideas off each other. Don't be afraid to think outside the box. When you've got at least three possible solutions for each stressor, then think about what can be applied practically and what might be the best option. Then cross out all the ones that simply won't work or couldn't be used. While they may not be useable at this point, they helped you creatively design the 'real' solutions and may still be useful if all else fails. From the remaining options, choose the three most useful and write them in order of preference into the right column of the table.

This action of taking control not only gives you options to reduce your stress but it also gives you confidence that you're a capable person who's able to take control of your life and situations that impact on you. The action of brainstorming creative ideas helps your brain to see that it really does has the power and capability to categorise issues and bring about suitable solutions. Creative brainstorming does more than just give us the solutions, it empowers us to see alternatives ways of dealing with issues that may have seemed insurmountable earlier. This is an incredibly useful technique for opening up ideas and alternatives you never realised you were capable of achieving.

Stressors I can eliminate or control	Techniques to overcome them.		
	1		
	2		
	3		
	1		
	2		
	3		
	1		
	2		
	3		
	1		
	2		
	3		
	1		
	2		
	3		
	1		
	2		
	3		
	1		
	2		
	3		
	1		
	2		
	3		

Figure 13 Controlling Stressors Plan

Better Ways to Deal with Stress

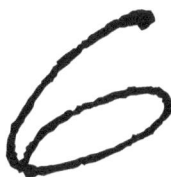

He who has health has hope; and he who has hope has everything (Arab proverb)

In this chapter, we're going to start working on the stressors that you can't eliminate or reduce. These are the ones you must find more creative and internally resourceful ways to deal with because they can't be avoided. Here we talk about a number of different techniques and approaches you can take that might help you deal with those uncontrollable stressors.

There are so many factors that are different for each of us and these will determine what techniques or approaches will work for you. Some of the things you may need to consider when trying these options are;

- Your workplace environment
- Your workplace culture
- Safety or shift restrictions
- Your personal preference
- The types of stressor you're facing
- Whether your reactions are physical, psychological or behavioural

However, before choosing a set of specific ways to deal with your stress, it's important to have a clearer understanding of your ability to control your situation and how you deal with each event.

Respond or React – Your Choice

In almost everything we do, either at work, with our families, with our friends or alone, we have the right to choose who we are and how we respond.

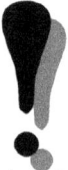

Important Note

It's important to remember that although you may not have control over the circumstances or events that you're in, you *always* have control over how you respond to them. You can choose to *respond* or *react* and it's all about the choices you make in terms of your situation specific management decisions.

Take Note

Responding

When you're faced with a difficult set of circumstances, if you choose to *respond,* you remain in control of yourself and increase your chances of a successful outcome. You remain the master of your life and you continue to be top of things. Your choices aren't random but rather they're controlled, predictable and well thought out. This stable, justifiable response enables you to make rational choices and take considered and positive steps towards more productive results.

This response comes from the rationality of your brain.

Reacting

By comparison, when you *react* to a situation, you lose all the control and you work from instinct or from a historical set of ingrained behaviours. You've probably conditioned yourself to deal with events in a certain way and when faced with a repeat of the event, you go into automatic pilot. This reaction takes away all the power and control and leaves you with no choices. In effect, the event is in control and you're just a slave to the process. This reaction comes from your raw emotions.

Armed with that information, one of your first and foundation options can be to make a conscious decision to respond to situations rather than react to them. This mean you take control and make sound choices that allow you to govern your own life rather than have it governed for you by unknown factors. While that sounds easy, how does it actually happen?

Put simply, by reading through the options in the next chapter and giving some a try, you're taking the first step to responding rather than reacting. You've made a conscious choice to be the controller and that's a powerful tool in your defence arsenal. Now let's see what ammunition you can use.

Proven Techniques to Deal with Stress

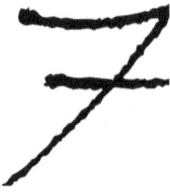

7

> *Better to light a candle than to curse the darkness. (Chinese Proverb)*

In this chapter, we're going to cover some of the most useful techniques and tools for dealing with stress. These techniques are recommended by counsellors, psychologists, rehabilitation specialists and occupational health and safety advisors throughout Australia and the world.

Reframe Your Stress

By believing you're stressed, you're letting yourself be a victim to that stress. This means that you're in effect giving control to something else and not allowing yourself to control it. You're reacting instead of responding. Instead, reframe your thoughts by telling yourself that you're simply reacting to difficult circumstances and that in fact you can control both the reactions and the circumstances that are contributing to your stress.

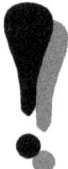

Take Note

Important Note

You are not your stress. It's external to who you are and a separate entity from you. This means looking at what's happening and taking responsibility for who you are and what happens to you by seeing stress as an outside factor you can deal with rather than considering it part of your personal makeup.

Figure 14 shows what happens when you fall into the reaction pattern associated with victimisation. With this mindset, you're controlled by the stress because you allow that to happen. Follow the steps in this illustration to see how your thoughts and subsequent actions can develop if you're not in control of how you think.

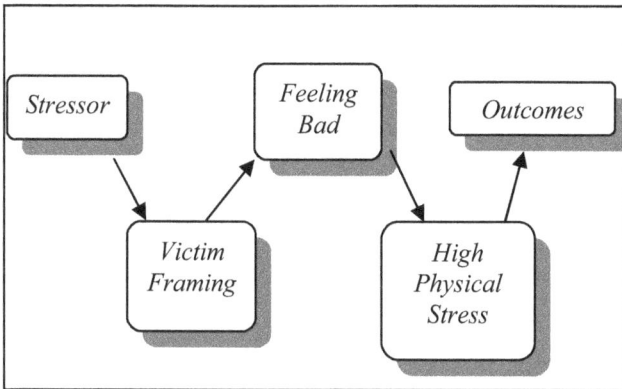

Figure 14 Victim Approach

Stressor
This is the circumstance that may be perceived as being a problem. For example: An important project deadline is approaching.

Victim Framing
This is how you might interpret the stressor. For example: "I'll never get this done in

time. Why did I get lumped with this job? I can't handle all this work". You're immediately allowing the stressor to engulf you and giving control to the situation rather than retaining it for yourself.

Feeling Bad

As a result of framing the circumstances as something you can't control, you may experience negative feelings. Example: Anxiety, embarrassment, fear, frustration. Now you see the entire event as being negative.

High Physical Stress

Now the brain begins to interpret the events as a threat and orders the body to go into fight or flight response. Example: Your muscles tense up, your head aches, your neck hurts from leaning over a computer for too long, you get constipation from inactive digestive system and a back ache from poor posture.

Outcomes

You begin to *act* the way your thoughts decided you should act. Example: Instead of just thinking irritable thoughts, you now actually *become* irritable and snappy. The boss and your colleagues observe your behaviour and make decisions about you based on your reactions. This may result in the perception that you can't handle the role or project and therefore any future opportunities become more limited.

Now let's compare that with the probable outcome if you choose instead to respond rather than react.

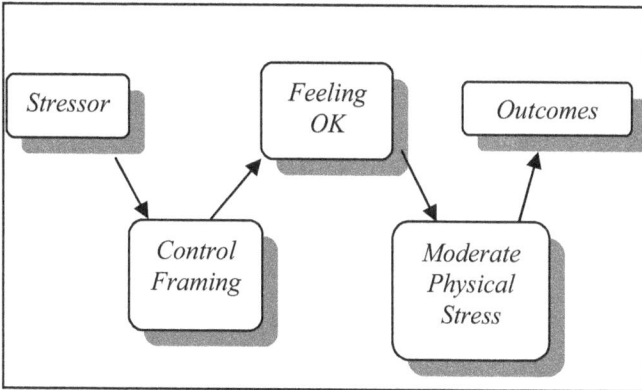

Figure 15 Control Approach

By responding, you're actively choosing to control the situation, your approach to it and you therefore have far greater control over the outcomes. This is a cognitive approach to the situation and is a means of changing the way you think about a situation and thus taking control. Figure 15 shows the steps in this process.

<u>Control Framing</u>

This is how you might interpret the stressor. For example: "This is a huge job but it can be done with a little planning. It's a good challenge for me to try and meet. What help do I need?" These thoughts place the control very firmly in your hands and give you a sense of power over the situation.

Feeling OK

As a result of framing the circumstances as something you can indeed control, you tend to experience more positive feelings about the situation. Give yourself permission to feel things in a more positive light and encourage yourself to aim for more acceptable feelings. Example: You're motivated to succeed, motivated to seek appropriate support, satisfied with the level of stimulation, a little anxious but you know you have a wider range of support options.

Moderate Physical Stress

Because your feelings are not perceived as negative and the circumstances are no longer personally threatening, the physical stress issues are reduced. Your body doesn't perceive the situation as a personal threat and so doesn't go into the 'fight or flight' mode. The stress levels are appropriate and motivate you toward success. Example: Your muscles may moderately tense up and adrenalin may rise but only enough to power you through the process.

Outcomes

You begin to *act* the way you've decided you should act so the outcomes you design come to fruition. In other words, you become the architect of your own behaviour and results. Example: You see yourself as succeeding in a rewarding challenge. You win and your positive outlook and self control are perceived by others as a strength. This perception may be enough for the boss to see you as the prime choice for more rewarding projects or invitations for promotion.

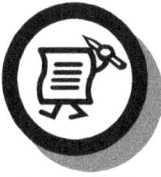

Thinking Using the Control Approach

Personal Task

Think of a recent occasion where you were affected by a stressor. It might be where you were asked to do some extra work or perhaps family life was difficult when your partner was unwell. Track your thoughts and actions through that process. Were they Victim or Control orientated?

Describe the stressor and what you thought about it

_____

_____

_____

_____

_____

_____

Was that Victim or Control thinking?

_____

_____

_____

_____

_____

_____

_____

How did you feel about the situation?

_____

_____

_____

_____

_____

_____

How did your feelings affect your thoughts?

_____

_____

_____

_____

_____

_____

_____

What physical response or reaction did you have to the situation?

_____

_____

_____

_____

_____

_____

_____

What was the outcome?

_____

_____

_____

_____

_____

_____

_____

Would you do anything differently next time? If so, what?

_____

_____

_____

_____

_____

_____

_____

See Your Doctor

With some positive thinking affecting your actions, it's also time to check your physical well being.

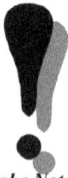

Important Note
If you're feeling overwhelmed by stress or if you're experiencing any physical symptoms that are worrying you in any way, you *must* consult your doctor or primary health care

Take Note

practitioner immediately.

Although stress can cause a variety of symptoms, they may also be the result of other illnesses. Better to be safe than sorry. Let your doctor know you're feeling stressed and ask their advice. They may be able to provide you with referrals to specialists or suggest consults with practitioners such as masseurs for muscle relaxation, psychologists for counselling or alternative practitioners such as acupuncturists, Chinese herbalists, Emotional Freedom Technique practitioners or naturopaths.

Make an Appointment to See Your Doctor

Although you've done a lot of work to diminish your stress and you might now have less physical symptoms, it's always wise to play it safe.

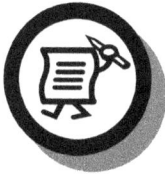

Personal Task

If you have any worrying symptoms at all, regardless how trivial you think they might be, make an appointment to see your doctor. Your doctor will become one of your greatest allies in beating the stress you face each day.

Employee Assistance Program (EAP)

Many organisations offer their staff free access to confidential Employee Assistance Programs or EAPs as they are known. These programs are usually paid for by the organisation but are operated by an external company who are staffed with qualified counsellors and psychologists. The idea behind EAPs is that where an employee may be affected by difficulties that may have a negative impact on their work, access to a qualified counsellor may often be all that's needed to overcome the problem.

EAPs are legally bound not to discuss your situation with anyone (unless of course you present as a risk of self harm or you intend to harm to others or conduct an illegal action). They're bound never to discuss your case with your employer and they only provide statistical information to the employer to aid them in financial accounting. Your name or any difficulties you're facing will not be given to the employer. You can seek help and support from an EAP for any problem regardless of whether you perceive it to be caused by work, home, relationships or any other element of your life. The service is usually free and in many instances you can attend during work hours or you may prefer to consult with your EAP outside work time.

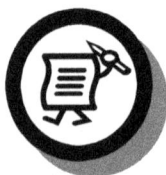

Personal Task

Check Your Access to an EAP
Find out from your Human Resource Manager or other appropriate officer if your employer provides an EAP service. If so, make a note of who they are and how you can contact them. Keep these details handy and use them if you need to. Two heads are often better than one when trying to solve issues.

The 'Quickie' Relaxation Technique

In her book, "Hiding What We Feel, Faking What We Don't", Sandi Mann offers a technique that can be used when you're too busy to stop but still need to take control of your stress levels. It's a simple three step process that enables you to regain control of your emotions and your body tension without anyone knowing what you're doing. Great for those times when you just want to scream at someone!

Step 1

Very often when we get stressed, we tense particular muscles in our bodies, often the neck and shoulders, and after a period of time this can cause headaches as well as aches and pains in other areas and general tiredness. The main problem with this is that we often don't even realise these muscles are tensed and so we continue to stress them.

Focus on the muscles in your hands and clench and then unclench them by making a fist. Do this three times quite slowly and in a focused fashion. Then tighten and relax the muscles in your arms three times slowly and carefully. Follow that by slowly tightening and relaxing the muscles in your legs three times and then lastly do the same with the muscles of your buttocks.

By taking a moment to really notice what your muscles are doing and actively and deliberately relaxing them, you can take control of your body's physical responses to stress and minimise the repercussions. Just the action of concentrating on your muscles and relaxing them again can be a real help and it only takes a minute or two to check.

Step 2

When the body is tense, the limb muscles use up more oxygen than normal as they get ready for a flight or fight response and so correct breathing to control oxygen intake is very important.

Notice your breathing. Take control by taking slow, deep breathes. With every breath out, try to imagine that you are blowing out all the negative feelings you are currently experiencing. This might be anger, frustration, sadness or boredom. With every breath out, the negative or destructive emotion is being pushed away. Now try to imagine that with every breath inwards, you're breathing in peacefulness. Do this exercise for a minute or two or until you feel more in control of your emotions.

Step 3

Take a closer look at your posture. Now that you're breathing more slowly and deeply and you're aware of the muscles in your body and they're more relaxed, how are you standing or sitting? Is your posture helping you relax or is it contributing to your aches and pains?

If you're sitting, notice your shoulders. Lower them back down again (they're probably hunched up) and then relax your legs. Lay your hands peacefully on your lap. Keep those shoulders loose and slightly slumped. If you're standing, make sure your feet are about a foot apart, uncross your arms, and lower your shoulders again. Take on more of an 'at ease' stance and deliberately focus your posture to a more relaxed rather than regimental approach.

Practicing the Quickie

You need not be stressed to practice this technique. In fact if get used to the process before you need it, you'll be much better prepared when you need it.

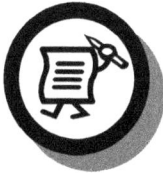

Personal Task

Find ten minutes today and a private place where you won't be disturbed and practice the three steps. Practice the technique three more times until you feel comfortable with it. Then you'll be ready to use it as needed without anyone knowing.

Displacement

Whenever you're feeling particularly angry or frustrated, it often helps to release that energy. That doesn't mean you can take out your anger on a colleague or a customer though! This technique allows you to channel that frustration and anger and direct it to a more suitable target like a stress ball or a punching pillow.

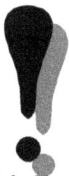

Important Note

It's always wise to use this technique in a private place where you can't be overheard, seen or disturbed. Other people may not realise you're yelling at, or punching a pillow and not

Take Note

another person! People also tend to get embarrassed and nervous at someone else's anger so spare them their worry and also the quizzical glances you might get and use this technique in a private location.

Go to your private place and take your target object with you. It might be a foam stress ball, a cushion, or even a rolled up towel will do. Make sure there's nothing in the room that might break if you throw things around. Think about the distressing event you've just been through and this time, instead of holding that anger or frustration in as you probably had to before, this time let it out. Think of your target object as the person or piece of equipment that made you feel so upset and really let them have it! Yell at your cushion, scream at the stress ball, and throw that towel at the wall, jump all over the pillow while you tell it what you think of it.

You can really go to town with this semi role playing technique. It's a great way of releasing all that anger, frustration or tears. It also ensures that your destructive feelings are not stored up to be later thrown at your spouse or children or some other unsuspecting, innocent person.

Reconstruct the Actions of Others

We've already looked at how you can reframe your own thoughts so that you have greater control over the outcomes. Now let's take that one step further and look at how you can reconstruct the actions of others when their behaviour causes you concern, worry, fear or anger.

Reconstructing the way we look at others helps us to see it in a different way and often enables us to respond quite differently. For instance, when you come across a rude, arrogant or abusive customer or even a colleague, instead of viewing them as rude and abusive, you could view them as someone with a problem that's making them behave the way they are. This slight change in your thoughts about them can help you remain calm enough to deal with their behaviour because you now see it as a symptom of some other, possibly unknown problem they are facing. Now rather than reacting equally as negatively as they are, you're probably more motivated to respond in a sympathetic or certainly more rational manner that helps resolve the situation rather than fuel it further.

Use self-talk to guide you through this. Keep saying something like, "this person has some real personal problems that's making them behave this way" so that you can keep your own actions on track. Talk nicely to yourself and remind yourself that you have the power and the strength to remain mature and in control. "I am a rational person who's always in control".

With practice, this technique works very well but every now and again, we have a bad day and things don't always go according to plan. If you don't quite get it right sometimes, don't beat yourself up about it. Think about the moment when you gave away the control and tell yourself that while you didn't quite keep it together that time, you know what happened and you know how to do it better next time. Be nice to yourself and congratulate yourself on your successes! Celebrate when you get it right and don't dwell on the times when you didn't quite get it right.

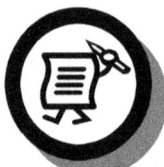

Reconstructing Practice
This technique takes a lot more practice than the previous ones. This is because you know yourself better than others and it's not always easy to think of reasons why someone else might be behaving the way they are. Never the less it's a good technique to master, particularly if you work in an area where you come up against a lot of angry or frustrated people.

Personal Task

Play Acting the Role

Although we're encouraged to 'be ourselves' rather than faking our responses, another way to cope with the stress created through dealing with difficult people, is to role play your way through the event as it's actually happening rather than replaying it afterwards as in the last exercise.

Imagine yourself as having two roles. Your personal being, the 'real' you is one. Another being is the role you play at work. It might be a receptionist, editor, boilermaker or office manager. That role is your 'workplace self'. Now take the real you and wrap it up in the workplace you. The real you, including your emotions, is now firmly and securely wrapped up and protected by the workplace you. Imagine all the negative accusations and behaviour thrown at you by the other person as just hitting and bouncing off the 'workplace you'. The 'real you' inside never gets touched by the angry words because it's safely cocooned inside the role you play at work. This technique helps you to deflect personal attacks from others and helps you to protect your inner self from the destructive words or actions of other, less thoughtful people.

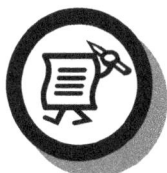

Drawing up Your Play Acting Sheet

Personal Task

One of the best ways to practice this technique is to draw it out on paper first and then keep it somewhere where you can look at it as you need to. Stick the sheet on a wall beside you or leave it in your drawer where you can see it frequently to remind you that you do have another coping technique up your sleeve. You need to always remind yourself about the two versions of yourself so that you can deflect any negativity off the 'workplace you' rather than the 'real you'.

Take a blank sheet of paper and either paste a photograph of yourself on it or draw a picture of yourself. A simple stick figure will be adequate as long as you can relate your 'real' self in the figure. Write the words "real me" underneath the photograph or drawing.

Now draw a circle all around the "real me" and write a note that shows that the circle is your "workplace me". Your workplace self will now be surrounding and protecting the real you. Have a look at the circled figure on the right of Figure 16 below.

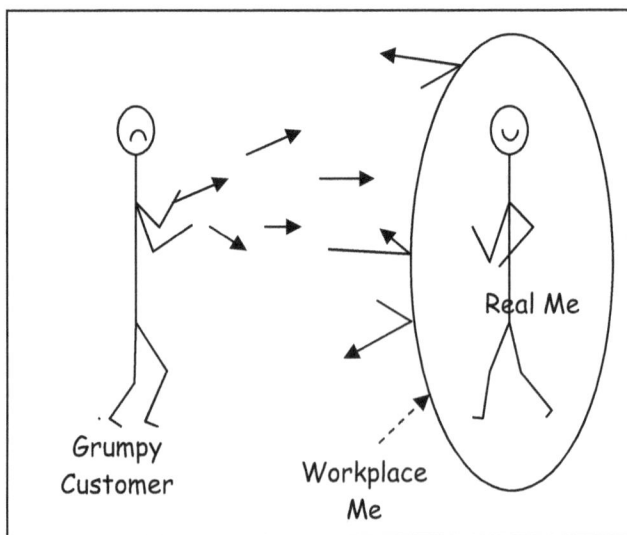

Figure 16 Play Acting the Role

If you've had any recent events where you've been criticised, abused, yelled at, or been negatively affected by a customer or colleague, you can incorporate this into your drawing. Draw a stick figure somewhere else on the paper and name them as the person who affected you. Then draw sharp arrows from them towards your workplace self but draw the arrows as bouncing back off the circle. This picture can become the representation of all that negative energy bouncing off your workplace role while the real you remains safe and protected.

Speak Nicely to Yourself

It's sad but all too often true that we don't speak very nicely to ourselves. What we say inside our heads to ourselves, our 'self-talk' is often very destructive and comes out of a condition I call the 'no syndrome'. Take a minute to think about the first word that most infants learn the meaning of pretty quickly. What do you think that word is? For most children, the word is, 'no".

"No, don't touch the stereo, you'll mess it up."
"No, leave that dog alone, it might bite you."
"John, I said no! You can't ride your bike to school, you're too young!"
"Look Katie, just because the other girls dye their hair doesn't mean you can – No!"

Eventually, after hearing this many years, that festers and develops into,

"Don't be ridiculous, you don't have the brains to do that university course."
"You'll never get that job, you don't have the skills."
"You are kidding! You want a loan to start a business? "No way, you haven't got what it takes."

Your brain hears all that, takes it on board, decides it's all fact and starts repeating it back to you as 'self-talk'. Eventually you hear yourself saying,

"I can't do this, I'm not good enough."
"I'll never be able to get this right."
"I'm just no good at any of this stuff."

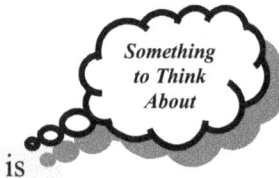

Something to Think About

What's happened to so many of us over the years is that we've listened to the 'no' sentences for too long. We've begun to believe what others have said about us. "I can't do anything." The very dangerous 'no syndrome' has turned into the even more dangerous, "no I can't because…" paradigm.

Because many of us were brought up in this "no you can't because…" paradigm, that's what we believe about ourselves. It's our role model for life, it's the way we see ourselves and the world. Because it's our only role model, we usually bring our children up the same way and the paradigm just keeps going.

This paradigm means we doubt our abilities and sometimes even talk ourselves out of achieving and succeeding before we've even started. Those gremlins eat away at our self confidence so that we question our abilities and when a stressor comes along and offers us even more challenges, very often, it all seems too much and we give up. We find excuses not to do things and achieve because it's easier than trying and maybe failing. The only problem with this is that perhaps had we given ourselves a chance, we might actually have achieved success!

Research shows that most of us won't accept a compliment or positive appraisal from someone until we've heard it eleven times! Yet we take on board any negative comments the very first time. That's an eleven to one ratio beating you up every day. No wonder we doubt ourselves so much!

One simple way to help is to learn to speak nicely to yourself in your head. Reframe that self-talk into a more positive paradigm so that you begin to focus and concentrate more on what you do well rather than on what you think you do badly. Make a list of all the things you know you are good at and that you are thankful for. Often this will be things you enjoy doing and events or activities that are special to you so it doesn't even have to be about work. The list might include;

When you have your list of successes, grow it. Add to it as you achieve more and celebrate it often. Look at it every day and remind yourself that you are special and that you don't need to be stuck in the "no I can't because..." paradigm. Don't make excuses for why you think you can't do something. Instead, give yourself reasons to say "yes, I can because…" and choose to live in that paradigm.

Driving	☑	Listening to others	☑
Gardening	☑	Being thoughtful and caring	☑
Writing	☑	Managing people	☑
Football	☑	Sticking to the job	☑
Carpentry	☑	Having fun with my kids	☑
Swimming	☑	Delegating tasks	☑
Fishing	☑	Motivating others	☑
Acting	☑	Setting targets	☑
Typing	☑	Solving problems	☑
Cooking	☑	Job hunting	☑

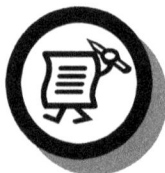

Personal Task

Drawing up Your List of Successes

It's time now for you to write down and celebrate all the things you're good at and thankful for. Many people find this task quite difficult because we've been trained from childhood to see what we do wrong rather than what we do right. Remember the 'no syndrome'? It's a powerful tool and a dangerous legacy that keeps us from seeing our real strengths.

In the table for this task at Figure 17, there are two columns. One is for all the things you do exceptionally well. It doesn't matter what these things are. The important thing is that they are *your* specialities. They're the things you can be proud of. The other column is for all the people, things, events, places, memories and anything else that you're especially grateful for. They are the things that make you smile.

Use a photocopy of Figure 17 (overleaf) so you always have the blank copy in this book to build. Then start writing on your own photocopy straight away. Keep it and stick it to your fridge because the more you see it, the more you can focus on your strengths and the more you can accept the wonderful person that you actually are but often deny. Add to your table as you find more things that you can celebrate about yourself. And celebrate big time over those successes! Pat yourself on the back for your gifts and strengths. They're what make you the special person you're growing into.

This activity might seem trivial or even vain but the fact remains that your self-talk determines who you actually are and it's really important to take control of the decisions about your successes and use them as the basis for your self-talk rather than the legacy of what came before.

My Special Skills	What I'm Thankful For

Figure 17 My Positive 'Self-talk'

Emotional Freedom Technique (EFT)

This technique is one of the 'energy field' techniques and isn't scientifically traditional at all as many other psychological tools are. Instead it's the marriage of western cognitive approaches and eastern energy principles.

Affectionately known by practitioners as emotional acupuncture, the technique involves tapping on particular pressure points while focusing on the negative issue or feeling. It can be used to control and usually treat in full all manner of unwanted emotions including those from phobias, past experiences and of course current stress. The resulting reduction in worry, anger, fear or any other destructive emotion is swift, often within minutes.

While it's a fairly new technique, but based on centuries of eastern knowledge and skill, research to date shows it's a powerful tool for the reduction and elimination of damaging emotions. The technique is simple to learn and there are qualified practitioners all over the world who are able to teach individuals how to take fast, effective control over limiting beliefs and destructive emotions.

To find out more about EFT, and to locate a local practitioner, log on to the web site http://www.emofree.com.

Twenty Minute Holiday

They say a change is as good a rest but when you're stuck at work all day or tied to the house all week long, it's hard to get a relaxing change into your day. One way to do it is to use the twenty minute holiday technique to fool your brain and body into thinking it's experienced a restful change. This technique is used in meditation and by relaxation advocates all over the world.

You can buy relaxation tapes and CDs and for the most part, they are all very good. One way to save a little money is to record yourself reading this story and then play it back each time you want to 'escape'.

Find yourself a warm, peaceful area where you won't be disturbed by noise or people. You're aiming for peace and tranquillity with this exercise. It's best done while lying on the floor although you can still relax very well with practice while seated. Be careful about doing this exercise while lying in bed though because it can put you to sleep. While that's great if it's late at night, it's not so good at 11.45am. If you're supposed to be back at work in half an hour, sleep may not be the result you were hoping for!

Get comfortable, close your eyes, relax and play the recording of this story letting yourself drift away with the words.

Make sure you're comfortably lying down or seated in a supportive, comfortable chair. Close your eyes and now notice your breathing. Slow your breathing down so it's rhythmical and calm. Take the air you breathe in right down into the base of your lungs. Breathe in and out slowly, focusing on your calm, relaxed and deep breaths in and out.

Now imagine you walking in a beautiful pasture. The field is full of lush grass and wild summer flowers. The birds are singing and the butterflies are dancing over the blossoms. The sun is bright and warm and soothing. It bathes your body in peaceful warmth and light.

As you walk, you see in the distance a lovely stream that rambles throughout the meadows. It's gentle rippling sounds remind you of spring as it brings life to the lush green valleys. Walk towards the stream now and sense its peace.

You follow the path of the stream for a little while and you see fish swimming playfully. The water is crystal clear and fresh. Slowly, the stream widens until it becomes a small river. It's still gentle and running smoothly. Up ahead you see a few small boats. There's a little sailing boat and some dinghies and a couple of rowing boats. They're all just nestling peacefully in their moorings.

One of the boats belongs to you and you step into it and sit on the warm, smooth wooden seat. You untie its moorings and allow the river to gently guide you along its path. The boat lazily drifts through the water, gently swaying with the cool breeze. The sun shines down serenely and you drink in the peace and tranquillity. It's a glorious day as the birds sing around you, the water ripples below you and boat gently winds its way along the peaceful water.

Eventually, the boat arrives at a mooring and you carefully tie the rope to a pole to keep the boat safe. You step out of the craft onto dry land. The ground is firm below you. You are back in a wonderful meadow of thick clover and soft green grass. You can smell the fresh aroma of newly cut grass and it lifts your spirits.

It's been a beautiful day on the river but you realise that you must go back to what you were doing before you entered this journey. You walk across the meadow towards your real waiting world. It looks inviting, exciting and welcoming. You know that your peaceful journey along the river has been a wonderful way to prepare for the joy of your life. As you walk towards home, you begin to see what needs to be done and you can already see better ways of doing things and enjoying life.

Now slowly open your eyes. Take notice of your breathing again. Keep it nice and slow, calm and deep. When you are ready, get up carefully and begin the process of the rest of your day.

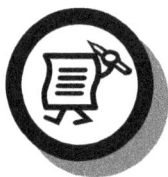

Taking Your Twenty Minute Holiday Successes

To save you money and shopping time, you can always make your own copy of this peaceful relaxation story.

Personal Task

Simply find a blank CD and record yourself reading the story. When you read it, do so slowly and calmly. You might be surprised how quickly you talk even when you've told yourself to slow down.

Innovative Coping Methods

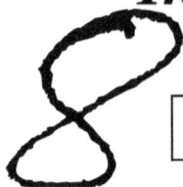

8

A journey starts with a single step

Just as there are limitless stressors and reactions to stress, so are there countless ways in which you can help your body rebalance and stabilise itself so that it can better deal with stress.

One of the greatest things you can do to prevent stress becoming a negative impact is to ensure you have a well balanced life where time with family, social activities, hobbies and relaxation have as much importance and emphasis in your life as work. These refreshing and energising activities regenerate the body's batteries and enable you to more effectively deal with stress. Because we're all different, some of the ideas here may not appeal to you while you may find others inspiring and motivating. The secret is to try those strategies that you think might work for you and see what happens!

Yoga	Meditation
Massage	Bush walking
Fishing	Pilate's
Painting	Cycling
Reiki	Screaming
Praying	Laughing
Wood turning	Dress making

Story writing	Cooking
Bird breeding	Sailing
Horse riding	Candle making
Do a TAFE class	Camping
Singing	Photography
Amateur drama	Volunteer work
Tai Chi	Mechanics
Garden weeding	Internet chat room
Clay modelling	Swimming
Indoor cricket	Teach your skill

Your List of Regeneration Activities

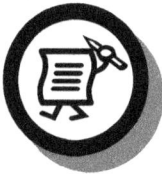

Personal Task

The list on the previous page might not include activities that suit your lifestyle or that even appeal. Spend some time now writing down all the things you love doing and that rejuvenate you. Include in the list your hobbies and the fun things you love to do alone or with family and friends. Use this list as your battery re-charger.

About the Author

Ziggy has been designing and facilitating workshops and training programs on stress and other subjects for over twenty years. Her expertise is recognised across Australia and she is frequently asked to design and implement professional development in the fields of:

- De-stressing the workplace
- Coaching to increase the value of skills development
- Using body language to gain better results with other people
- Improving communication techniques

With a plethora of qualifications including a Doctorate in which she developed a new theory of learning, a Masters Degree in Professional Education and Training, a Bachelors Degree in Psychology, a Diploma in Training & Assessment Systems, and a Diploma in Frontline Management, she's also been a Director on the national, governing board of Australia's premier professional development group, the Australian Institute of Training and Development and in the year 2000 she won the coveted WA Information Technology Micro Business of the Year.

Ziggy balances her busy and successful career by teaching students in her much loved religion, continuing to adore her four wonderful, grown up children and writing.

Further Reading

Adams, J. (1998) Stress: A friend for life. The C.W. Daniel Company Ltd.

Aslet, D. & Cartaino, C. (1997) Keeping Work Simple: Solutions for a Saner Workplace. Storey Books.

Berglas, S. (2001) Reclaiming the Fire: How Successful People Overcome Burnout. Random House.

Cameron-Hill, P. & Yates, S. (2000) You won't die laughing: How to have less stress in your life and more fun. Argyle Publications.

Cooper, C., Cartwright, S. (1997) Managing Workplace Stress. Sage Publications.

Davidson, J. (1999) The Complete Idiot's Guide To Managing Stress. Macmillan Publishing.

Davis, M., McKay, M., Eshelman, E. (2000) The Relaxation & Stress Reduction Workbook. New Harbinger Publications.

Gatto, R., (1993) Controlling Stress in the Workplace: How You Handle What Happens. Gatto Training Associates Press.

Lenson, B. (2002) Good Stress, Bad Stress: An Indispensable Guide to Identifying and Managing Your Stress. Marlowe & Co.

Mann, S. (1999) Hiding What We Feel, Faking What We Don't. Element Books.

Maslach, C., Leiter, M. (1997) The Truth About Burnout: How Organizations Cause Personal Stress and What to Do About It. Jossey-Bass.

McEwen, B., Lasley, E. (2002) The End of Stress As We Know It. Joseph Henry Press.

Montgomery, B. (1992) Coping with Stress. Pitman Publishing.

Potter, B., Frank, P. (1998) Overcoming Job Burnout: How to Renew Enthusiasm for Work. Ronin Publishing.

Quick, J., Nelson, D., Hurrell, J. (1997) Preventive Stress Management in Organizations. American Psychological Association.

Sapolsky, R. (1998) Why Zebras Don't Get Ulcers: An Updated Guide to Stress, Stress-Related Diseases, and Coping. W H Freeman & Co.

Seaward, B. (2002) Managing Stress. Jones & Bartlett Publishing.

Selye, H. (1978) The Stress of Life. McGraw-Hill Trade.

UK National Work-Stress Network. (2003) <u>What is Work-Related Stress?</u> http://www.worstress.net/whatis.htm

Victoria State Government. (2003) <u>Better Health Channel</u>. http://www.betterhealth.vic.gov.au

Wells, S., Lake, D. (2001) <u>Pocket Guide to Emotional Freedom</u>. Waterford Publishing.

Wilke, W. (1995) <u>Understanding stress breakdown</u>. Millennium Books.

Index

Your Notes

www.ingramcontent.com/pod-product-compliance
Lightning Source LLC
Chambersburg PA
CBHW031522270326

41930CB00006B/481